The Clean Eating Ultimate Cookbook And Diet Guide!

Clean Eating

Low Fat, Paleo, And Low Carb Recipes For Maximum Weight Loss And To Boost Your Metabolism For Fast Results!

Sarah Brooks

Copyright © 2014 Sarah Brooks

STOP!!! Before you read any further....Would you like to know the Secrets of Body Transformation?

If your answer is yes, then you are not alone. Thousands of people are looking for the secret to rapidly burn body fat, keep the weight off, become healthier, and truly transform their body and life for good.

If you have been searching for these answers without much luck, you are in the right place!

Not only will you gain incredible insight in this book, but because I want to make sure to give you as much value as possible, right now for a limited time you can get full **100% FREE access to a VIP bonus EBook** entitled **THE 7 KEYS TO BODY TRANSFORMATION!**

Just Go Here For Free Instant Access:

www.liveFitVIP.com

Legal Notice

Disclaimer Notice

Table Of Contents

Introduction

I want to thank you and congratulate you for purchasing the book, *"Clean Eating: The Clean Eating Ultimate Cookbook And Diet Guide! – Low Fat, Paleo, And Low Carb Recipes For Maximum Weight Loss And To Boost Your Metabolism For Fast Results!"*

This book contains proven steps and strategies on how to lose weight and boost your metabolism as quickly as possible based on the principles of clean eating and using popular diet recipes like low fat, paleo, and low carb recipes.

These days, you need to be more mindful of the kinds of food that you eat. You have to make sure that what you are eating is as natural as possible to provide you with the essential nutrients that your body needs without worrying about side effects or acquiring diseases. People these days choose convenience over health by buying processed and ready-to-eat foods that do not contribute much to your health. In this fast paced world where fast food and instant meals are popular, you have to be more disciplined with the meals that you cook not only for yourself but also for your whole family. This book will give you some basic facts and background on the principles of clean eating and different kinds of diet plans and strategies like low fat, paleo, low carb, carb cycling, flexible, and IIFYM. You can also find some tips on how to lose maximum weight, boost your metabolism, and get in shape. To get you started on your clean eating diet plan, you can use the recipes provided in the last few chapters of this book.

Thanks again for purchasing this book, I hope you enjoy it!

Chapter 1: Clean Eating Cookbook And Diet Guide

You have probably heard of clean eating from one of your health conscious or diet enthusiast friends. If not, you are probably asking the question that many people are asking, what exactly is clean eating? The main concept of clean eating is eating foods at their most natural state. This includes foods that are raw, fresh, and unprocessed. It is not just about the quantity but more on the quality of food that you eat. Clean eating is not just a diet fad or trend. It is a sound approach to healthy living through eating the right kinds of food that gives you the energy you need and makes you a healthier individual.

If you are going to adopt clean eating in your lifestyle, you need to understand its basic principles.

Eat whole and natural foods

Whole and natural foods are foods that have not been processed and are usually packed in a box, can, and plastic packaging. A bag of fresh beans may be packed in a plastic bag but this does not mean that these beans are not whole or natural. It is important that the foods that you eat are fresh or are in their most natural state, which means less cooking and very little processing, if at all.

Add fat, carbohydrate, and protein to your diet

Good fat and carbohydrate are essential minerals and they are easy to get from the usual foods that you eat everyday like grains, oil, pasta, and so on. However, many people lack protein in their diet, especially breakfast. It is important to get the right amount of protein that your body needs to help develop your muscles and also make you feel full longer.

Eat small meals frequently

The clean eating diet advises you to eat about five to six small meals in a day. This includes the usual breakfast, lunch, and dinner, plus two to three snacks in between meals. By eating small meals frequently, you will not go hungry easily which can often lead to overeating or eating just about anything you can grab. The small meals throughout the day also help stabilize the level of sugar in your bloodstream which prevents energy lag.

Drink at least two liters of water per day

This will keep your body hydrated which will prevent you from feeling tired. Avoid high calorie drinks like soda or energy drink because you need to get your calories from the food that you eat and not your drinks. It is also important to use a reusable canteen rather than plastic.

Learn how to read labels

Clean eating requires you to learn how to read labels because this is where you will find the ingredients. If the list of ingredients contain long names that are difficult to pronounce, this could mean that it has an artificial ingredient which is banned from clean eating.

Chapter 2: Low Fat Diet—An Overview

If you want to lose weight and boost your metabolism, you should incorporate some popular diet plans in your clean eating lifestyle like the popular low fat diet.

What is the low fat diet?

Everyone knows that foods with high fat content can make you gain weight. This is because fats have more calories than other nutrients or minerals. One gram of fat provides nine calories, which is more than twice the amount of calories that protein or carbohydrate provide (each provides four calories per gram). Low fat diet, like the South Beach diet, restricts your fat consumption not only to lose weight but to prevent certain diseases like obesity and heart disease. If you reduce fat in your diet, you are automatically cutting back on calories which make it easier for you to lose weight. This also allows you to eat more food without adding more calories.

It is recommended that an average adult should only get about 20% to 35% of their recommended daily calorie intake from fats—the rest should be from other sources. This means that if you are on a 2,000-calorie diet, you should only get about 44 to 77 grams of fat per day.

What foods to eat and what to avoid

You need to avoid high fat foods like regular whole milk, dairy products, pasta, meat and meat products, poultry with skin, baked treats, sweets, nuts, oils, mayonnaise, margarine, and so on. You may think that there too many foods to avoid which might make it difficult for you to follow this diet. However, you need to remember that almost all of the foods these days have low fat alternatives.

When you go to the grocery, you should buy low fat food items instead of their regular counterparts such as buying low fat or fat-free milk and dairy products, low fat cold cuts, lean meat, skinless poultry, fish, and other low fat food substitutes. Instead of adding avocado slices to your sandwich, you should instead add slices of cucumber. Instead of preparing pasta in white sauce or alfredo, you should instead prepare whole wheat pasta in marinara sauce.

It is also important to choose a healthier way of cooking your food such as baking, broiling, steaming, and grilling instead of frying. If you need to fry or sauté foods, you should use a non-stick pan to limit the amount of oil that you need to use. You can also use nonstick cooking spray instead of oil.

Chapter 3: Paleo Diet—An Overview

The Paleo diet, which is short for the Paleolithic diet, is diet plan that tries to imitate the diet of humans who lived in the Paelolithic area, which is mostly composed of wild plants and animals. This diet encourages followers to eat foods that have been available to human at that time, including processed foods and domesticated plants and animals for human consumption. Proponents of this diet fad claim that modern humans were not able to adapt to the fast change in their diet when agriculture was invented. They claim that modern humans are still best adapted to the original diet of ancient people, making it easier for them to digest the kind of food that our ancestors eat and prevent modern day diseases.

The diet

The Paleo diet is high in protein. Proponents of this diet believe that our ancestors had 19% to 35% calories from protein. It is also lower in carbohydrates and salt but higher in fiber. It also has a moderate to high fat content which are mostly good fats like omega 3, polyunsaturated, and monosaturated fats. Unhealthy fats are also avoided like trans-fat and omega 6 fats.

What foods to eat and what not to eat

The foods that you can eat if you are on a Paleo diet are lean meat, fruits and berries, non-starchy vegetables, nuts, and honey. Refined sugar is banned from this diet because people from the Stone Age, which also refers to the Paleolithic era, did not have refined sugar in their diet. If you want to sweeten up your food, you can add raw honey instead. The diet allowed very little dairy food, grains, and salt. Some even completely ban these foods from their diet. Dairy products involve modern ay processing while cereal grains are a result of agriculture, which is another modern discovery. Modern diets are high in salt, which is why the Paleo diet recommends foods with low sodium content.

Benefits

You might think that it is not a good idea to have the same diet as our ancestors who lived short and brutal lives. However, you cannot deny that this diet plan has a lot of health benefits, such as weight loss, stable blood sugar, balanced energy, improved immunity, and anti-inflammatory benefits. This diet plan may be difficult to follow for some people but it can still be beneficial because it prevents you from eating processed foods, sweets, and other foods that usually cause diseases.

Chapter 4: Low Carb Diet—An Overview

Just like the low fat diet, this diet limits the consumption of a certain nutrient, in this case, carbohydrates. There are a number of low carb diets that become popular over the years, such as the Atkins diet and the South Beach diet. It is based on the premise that low carbohydrate consumption can lead to low insulin production. This in turn can result to your body using the fats and protein stores as the main sources of energy, which helps people lose weight.

This diet is also called ketogenic diet because a person undergoes ketosis when carbohydrate consumption is lowered. This is a state where the body produces ketone substances that are used by other body parts which cannot use fat as a source of energy, like your brain and red blood cells. A diet low in carbohydrate helps treat obesity and diabetes.

Why low carb diet?

For many people, the easiest and most effective way to lose weight is to go on a low carb diet. This is because blood sugar levels increase when you eat foods that are rich in carbohydrates. And according to studies, the sugar level in your body plays an important role in weight loss.

Some experts and nutritionists do not agree with the low carb diet because they believe that a healthy diet should have the traditional sources of carbohydrates including grains like corn and wheat and vegetables like carrots and potatoes. These foods are rich in carbohydrates but they also provide other nutrients that the body needs, such as fiber.

What you can do to enjoy the benefits of a low carb diet is to find ways to lower your carbohydrate intake without sacrificing other nutrients. You can choose a variety of fruits, vegetables, and meat that are rich in other nutrients but have low carbohydrates. You also need to remember that this diet plan does not completely eliminate carbohydrate. It only promotes low carbohydrate intake that can help you lose weight and boost your metabolism.

Low carb food substitutes

Bread is a main staple in the Western diet. You can substitute low carb bread for regular bread or you can use other alternatives like low carb tortillas or high-fiber crisp breads. For pasta and noodles, you can use low carb pasta, spaghetti squash, or shirataki noodles. Some great substitutes for potatoes are mashed cauliflower or celery root called celeriac. There are so many low carb alternatives that you can use for cooking and preparing meals. All you need to do is to be creative and think outside the box.

Chapter 5: What Is Carb Cycling?

You also need to understand the term carb cycling that can help you lose weight and boost your metabolism. As the name implies, this diet alternates low to no carb diet with moderate to high carb diet. You are cycling your carbohydrate intake to achieve the best result. Proponents of this diet plan believe that completely eliminating carbohydrates or going on a low carb diet every day is not the ideal way to lose weight. They claim that low carbohydrate diet is only temporary. You still need to go back to a diet with adequate carbohydrate consumption to perform your daily functions properly.

How does it work?

The main purpose of cycling your carb intake is to give your body the energy that it needs and therefore boosting your metabolism and at the same time helping you to lose weight. The days are rotated among three types of carb days, low to moderate carb, high carb, and no carb days. Some people skip the no carb day because they believe that the body requires certain amount of carbohydrates every day.

What about protein and fats?

Protein consumption is the foundation of this type of diet. It is highly recommended to eat the right amount of protein that your body need every day. You need to know how much protein you should have in your every meal based on your weight and other factors. You should also observe consistent intake of dietary fats. During your low or no carb days, you should increase your fat intake because this is where you body will get its energy. You can lower your fat consumption on your moderate to high carb days.

Chapter 6: What Is Flexible Diet Or IIFYM?

Flexible dieting or IIFYM is another term that you need to know if you want to lose weight and boost your metabolism. You can still adopt clean eating if you are following the flexible diet or IIFYM concept. IIFYM stands for 'if it fits your macros'. 'Macros' refer to the three basic macronutrients that your body needs including protein, carbohydrate, and fat.

The flexible diet or IIFYM is not simply a diet trend but a concept. Instead of limiting certain food groups in your diet, you are allowed to eat anything healthy as long as it fits your macros. This is a looser diet concept compared to other diet plans that have a stricter structure and set of rules.

Flexible eating does not mean you can eat any kinds of foods as long as it meets your daily nutrient requirements. You should not get your carbohydrates and fats from burgers, fries, potato chips, ad pop tarts. These are not only junk foods but they will also not provide you with your protein needs, which means that you still need to get your protein from other food sources, like meat.

The main idea behind this diet plan is that your diet is more flexible than those that require you to eat only a certain kind of food at certain times of the day. You are encouraged to eat healthy and wholesome foods that are generally good for your health but it is okay if you eat sweets and chips from time to time or skip breakfast as long as you get your macronutrients from other meals of the day.

Many people prefer this kind of dieting because they do not feel deprived. They do not need to do major changes in their eating patterns and habits except for making sure that they meet the daily macronutrient requirement.

Chapter 7: How To Achieve Maximum Weight Loss, Boost Metabolism, And Get In Shape

Losing weight, boosting your metabolism, and getting in shape go hand in hand. The steps that you need to do to lose weight are the same steps that you need to do to boost your metabolism and get in shape and vice versa. With all the information that has been provided about different diet plans and concepts in the previous chapter, you now have a better idea how to improve your diet and eating habits. Here are some tips and advice for losing weight, boosting your metabolism, and getting in shape.

Find the right diet plan that will give you the most benefits

Clean eating is definitely a great diet plan because it puts more value on the quality of food that you eat. You cannot go wrong with eating natural foods with no artificial ingredients and have not undergone processes that can alter their nutritional value. At least everyone can agree to this. However, you can incorporate other diet plans with your clean eating lifestyle to get the maximum benefits. For example, you have to make sure that you meet your macronutrient requirements from the clean foods that you eat. You can also eat foods that are low in saturated fats. The key here is to adopt the good practices from each diet plan and incorporate them in your clean eating lifestyle.

Be more physically active

You need to have the right kind of exercise that can help you lose weight, boost metabolism, and get in shape. For instance, exercises that can help you build muscle such as weight lifting is essential for improving your metabolism and shedding a few extra pounds that will make your body more fit and toned. Each pound of muscle in your body burns about 6 calories per day, compared to fat which only burns 2 calories per pound per day.

Drink plenty of water

Water is essential for losing weight because it flushes out toxins from your body and helps you digest your food better. It also makes you feel fuller. Water also does wonder for your metabolic rate. Dehydration slows down your metabolic rate. If you drink enough water or other unsweetened beverage throughout the day, your body will remain hydrated which will improve your metabolism. You can also add water to your body by snacking on fresh fruits and vegetables rather than dry snacks like pretzel or chips.

Consult your doctor

Before changing anything in your diet, you first need to consult your doctor especially if you have special health conditions like diabetes or if you are overweight. This will help you choose the right diet plan that will be most beneficial to you and the kind of physical exercises that you need to do.

To help you get started on your clean eating lifestyle, you can check out the following recipes that are based on low fat, Paleo, and low carb diet plans that can help you lose weight and boost your metabolism.

Chapter 8: Low Fat Recipes

Banana Breakfast Smoothie

Ingredients:

- ½ cup 1% low fat milk
- 1 tbsp honey
- 1 large ripe banana, frozen and sliced
- 1 cup 2% reduced-fat plain Greek yogurt
- ½ cup crushed ice
- 1/8 tsp ground nutmeg

Instructions:

1. Using a powerful blender or food processor, blend in the milk, banana, honey, ice, and nutmeg until smooth and creamy.
2. Add the yogurt into the mixture and blend to mix it well.
3. Makes 2 servings.

Nutritional information (per serving):

Calories- 212, Fat- 3.6g, Carbohydrate- 34.2g, Protein- 14.2g, Fiber- 2g, Cholesterol- 9mg, Iron- 0.3 mg, Sodium- 75Mg, and Calcium: 200mg.

One-Pot Salmon with Snap Peas and Rice

Ingredients:

- 1 lb salmon fillet, skin removed
- 1 cup long-grain white rice
- 4 oz sugar snap peas, trimmed
- 4 scallions, trimmed and sliced
- 1/3 cup low-sodium soy sauce
- 1 tbsp dark brown sugar
- 1 tbsp grated ginger
- 2 tbsp rice vinegar
- Kosher salt and pepper to taste

Instructions:

1. Boil the white rice with water in a medium-sized skillet. Lower heat once the water is boiling and cover the skillet. Simmer for 10 minutes.
2. Make 4 diagonal slices of salmon of about 3/4 –inch thick and season with Kosher salt and pepper according to your liking. Place the seasoned salmon fillets on top of the rice while still simmering. Cover the skillet and cook for another 7 minutes.
3. While the rice and salmon are still cooking, add the snap peas on top. cover. Put the lid back on and cook for about 3 to 5 minutes, or until the salmon is opaque and flaky and the rice and peas are cooked enough.
4. Make the sauce by mixing the soy sauce, vinegar, sugar, and ginger in a small bowl. Pour a small amount over the salmon.
5. Makes 4 servings.

Nutritional information (per serving):

Calories- 418, Calories from fat- 19%, Fat- 9g, Saturated fat- 1g, Protein- 32g, Carbohydrate- 49g, Fiber 2g, Sugars- 5g, Sodium, 706mg, and Cholesterol- 72mg.

Multigrain Pasta with Leeks and Sweet Potatoes

Ingredients:

- 12 oz multigrain penne
- 3 leeks, cut into half moons
- 2 small or about 1 lb sweet potatoes, peeled and cut into bite-sized pieces
- 3 cloves garlic, minced
- ¾ cup Parmesan cheese, grated
- ¼ cup fresh sage, chopped
- ¼ tsp ground nutmeg
- Salt and pepper

Instructions:

1. Cook the pasta by following the instruction on the package. Drain the water but set aside ½ cup for cooking later.
2. Using a large skillet, heat the oil over medium heat. Add the leeks and cook for 4 minutes or until tender. Add the

sage and garlic and cook for 2 minutes or until fragrant. Add the sweet potatoes and salt and pepper to taste. Cook until about 6 to 8 minutes or until sweet potatoes are soft. Add ½ cup cheese and the water that you set aside. Let it simmer for about 4 minutes.

3. Add the nutmeg and the cooked penne pasta.
4. Divide among 4 bowls and sprinkle the remaining cheese. Makes 4 servings.

Nutritional information (per serving):

Calories- 541, Calories from fat- 22%, Fat-13g, Saturated fat- 0g, Carbohydrate 107g, Fiber- 12g, Protein- 26g, Sugars- 15g, Cholesterol- 13mg, and Sodium- 465mg.

Pop Corn Snack Bars

Ingredients:

- 8 cups plain popped popcorn
- ½ cup unsweetened shredded coconut
- ¾ cup almonds, chopped
- 2 cups rolled oats
- ½ cup dried apricots, thinly sliced
- ½ cup raisins
- ¾ cup honey
- ¾ cup light brown sugar, tightly packed
- ¼ tsp salt

Instruction:

1. Preheat oven to 350 degrees F. Put the shredded coconut on an ungreased baking sheet, making sure that they are evenly layered. Bake about 5 minutes and stir once or twice while baking. Transfer in a small bowl and set aside.
2. On the same baking sheet, spread the almonds evenly and bake for about 5 to 7 minutes or until fragrant an golden brown and stir once or twice while baking. Pour the almonds into the bowl with coconut shreds and set aside.
3. Spray a baking dish with cooking spray. Mix oats, popcorn, almonds, coconut, apricots, and raisins in a large bowl.
4. Cook honey, sugar, and salt in a small pan over low heat. Stir until sugar dissolves. Pour honey and popcorn

mixtures into the pan. Stir until all there are no dry spots and everything is well-coated.

5. Transfer the mixture into the baking dish and firmly press with your hands.

6. Put the dish in the fridge for 30 minutes and cut it into 24 bars.

Nutritional information (per bar):

Calories- 128, Fat- 3g, Saturated fat- 1g, Carbohydrate- 26g, Protein- 2g, Fiber- 2g, and Sodium- 26g.

Chapter 9: Paleo Diet Recipes

Chicken and Broccoli

Ingredients:

- 6 chicken breasts
- Lemon pepper and salt to taste
- 1 cup fresh broccoli

Instructions:

1. Choose the 'broil' setting in your oven and arrange rack in such a way that it is closer to the heat source.
2. Wrap a baking pan with aluminum foil. Set aside.
3. Use lemon pepper and sea salt to season the both sides of the chicken breasts.
4. Put the chicken breasts on the pan and broil until the bottom is golden or about 13 minutes.
5. Flip the chicken breasts and broil for another 12 minutes. Remove from the oven once both sides are golden.
6. To cook broccoli florets, put them in a pot of boiling water with cover. Remove until broccoli florets are tender enough.
7. Serve the chicken with your broccoli florets. Makes 6 servings.

Nutritional information (per serving):

Calories- 174, Total Fat 1.5g, Total Carbohydrate- 14g, and Protein 28g.

Sweet Potato Hash with Egg and Coconut Almond Waffle

Ingredients (Sweet Potato Hash with Egg):

- 1 organic egg
- ¼ sweet potato, shredded
- 1/8 tsp cayenne pepper
- 1/8 tsp garlic powder
- 1/8 tsp onion powder

- Coconut oil spray
- Sea salt and freshly ground pepper to taste

Instructions:

1. Coat skillet with coconut spray. Over medium heat, cook shredded sweet potato on the skillet for about one minute.
2. Add garlic powder, cayenne pepper, and onion powder and cook for another minute or two.
3. Add the egg once the sweet potatoes are starting to turn golden brown on the edges. Let the egg cook with the cover on.

Ingredients for Coconut-Almond Waffle:

- ¼ cup coconut, shredded
- 1 ½ cups almond flour
- 2 eggs
- ½ tsp baking soda
- 1 tbsp raw honey
- ¼ cup coconut milk in can
- 1 tsp vanilla extract
- Fresh raspberries
- Coconut flakes

Instructions:

1. Mix all the ingredients in a bowl.
2. Turn on the waffle maker and pour the mixture. Wait for the device to beep.
3. Once waffles are cooked, top with fresh raspberries and coconut flakes. You can add honey for added sweetness.

Nutritional information (for a full meal serving):

Calories- 583.19, Total Fat- 38.69g, Total Carbohydrate- 38.77g, and Protein 21.48g.

Artichoke and Healthy Ice Cream

Ingredients for the artichoke and sauce:

- 2 artichokes, remove stem and top of leaves
- 3 eggs, hard-boiled
- 2 tbsp green onions, finely diced

- 1 tsp mustard
- 1 tsp olive oil
- 2 tbsp white vinegar
- 3 tbsp water
- Sea salt and freshly ground pepper

Instructions:

1. Boil artichoke in a large pot filled with water for 45 minutes.
2. While waiting for the artichokes to cook, separate the egg yolks from the white. Slice the egg whites and smash the yolks with your fork.
3. Put the eggs in the bowl and add the remaining ingredients. Mix well.
4. Serve cooked artichokes with the egg sauce. Makes 2 servings.

Ingredients for the ice cream:

- 1 can coconut milk
- 1 sweet potato, skin removed and baked
- 2 egg yolks
- 1 tbsp maple syrup
- 2 tbsp cinnamon
- 1 tsp vanilla extract
- 1/8 tsp sea salt
- 1.8 tsp nutmeg

Instructions:

1. Leave the ice cream attachment in the freezer overnight.
2. In a food processer, puree the baked sweet potato and coconut milk.
3. Once smooth and thick, add cinnamon, nutmeg, vanilla, sea salt, and egg yolks. Process until smooth and creamy.
4. Refrigerate mixture for at least two hours.
5. After two hours or so, put the mixture in the ice cream maker and let it churn for about half an hour.
6. Makes 4 servings.

Nutritional information (per serving of both recipes):

Calories- 536.6, Total Fat- 36.2g, Total Carbohydrate- 36.5g, and Protein—22.64g.

Chapter 10: Low Carb Recipes

Granola Oatmeal Cereal

Ingredients:

- 3 cups old-fashioned cooking oats
- ½ cup SPLENDA
- 2 egg whites
- 1 tsp cinnamon
- ½ tsp salt
- ½ tsp baking powder
- ¼ cup canola oil

Instructions:

1. Preheat oven to 350 degrees F.
2. Mix oats, baking powder, cinnamon, salt, and Splenda in a mixing bowl.
3. Mix egg whites and canola oil in another bowl.
4. Combine both mixtures and bake for half an hour.
5. Makes 6 servings.

Nutritional information (per serving):

Calories- 259, Fat- 12g, Saturated fat- 1.5g, Carbohydrate- 30g, Protein- 7.7 g, Cholesterol- 0g, Sodium- 214mg, and Fiber- 4.5g.

African Chicken Stew

Ingredients:

- 1 lb chicken breasts, skinless, boneless, and cut into 2-inch pieces
- 1 tbsp water
- 1 tbsp garlic, minced
- 1 tbsp ginger, grated
- 1 tsp oregano, dried
- 1 Spanish onion, half minced and half chopped
- 1 28 oz can tomatoes with juices
- 1 habanero chili pepper, chopped

- 1/3 cup reduced-fat peanut butter
- ¼ cup ketchup
- 1 dash salt
- 1 dash pepper
- Canola cooking spray

Instructions:

1. Put the chicken in a resalable plastic bag. In a small bowl, mix the oregano, ginger, garlic, and water. Add this mixture inside the bag with chicken and massage. Once chicken breasts are fully coated, refrigerate overnight or for 6 hours.
2. Coat a Dutch oven with cooking spray and sear chicken until all pieces are white on all sides. Put them on the plate and set aside.
3. Coat the Dutch oven again with cooking spray and sauté onions, tomatoes with half the juice, ketchup, and chili pepper. Bring to a boil, then simmer for 10 minutes. Using a wooden spoon, break up the tomatoes into small pieces to bring out the juice.
4. Mix together peanut butter and remaining half of tomato juice and add to the pot. Add the cooked chicken and simmer for about 15 minutes.
5. Makes 4 servings.

Nutritional information (per serving):

Calories- 326, Fat- 9.8g, Saturated fat 2g, Carbohydrate- 27.6g, Protein- 34g, Fibe3- 4g, Calcium- 88mg, Sodium- 563mg, Cholesterol- 66mg, and Sugars- 14g.

Bagel Chips

Ingredients:

- 2 small bagels
- 2 tbsp canola oil
- 2 garlic cloves, crushed
- ¼ tsp dried mixed herbs
- ¼ tsp freshly ground black pepper

- ¼ tsp salt
- 1 oz Parmesan cheese, freshly grated

Instructions:

1. In a skillet, sauté the garlic and mixed herbs in hot oil for about one minute. Add the bagels in separate batches. Turn them until both sides are golden brown and crisp. Put the bagel chips on paper towels to absorb excess oil.
2. Season with salt and pepper and sprinkle with cheese.
3. Makes 6 servings.

Nutritional information (per serving):

Calories- 114, Fat- 7g, Carbohydrate- 10g, Protein- 3g, Calcium- 58mg, Sodium- 249mg, and Cholesterol 3mg.

Baked Trout

Ingredients:

- 4 trout fillets
- 1 tbsp whole wheat flour
- 1 tsp freshly grated lemon zest
- 1 tsp onion powder
- 2 tbsp parsley, chopped
- 1 lemon, cut into 8 thin slices

Instructions:

1. Preheat oven to 375 degrees F. Grease a baking sheet with cooking spray. Set aside.
2. Mix flour, onion powder, and lemon zest in a plastic or paper bag by shaking the bag. Add the trout fillets one at a time and coat with the mixture by shaking the bag. Place the coated trout fillets on the baking sheet. Brush the top of the fish with oil.
3. Bake the trout fillets for about 20 minutes or until fish is opaque. Once baked, put the fish on a plate and garnish with chopped parsley and 2 lemon slices for each fillet.
4. Makes 4 servings.

Nutritional information (per serving):

Calories- 221, Fat- 9.4g, Carbohydrate- 2.6g, Protein 30g, Calcium- 68mg, Sodium- 75mg, and Cholesterol- 82mg.

Lemonade

Ingredients:

- 7 ½ oz 100% fresh squeezed lemon juice or pure lemon juice from concentrate
- ¾ cup Equal sweetener
- 4 cups cold water
- 1 ice cube

Instructions:

1. Pour the lemon juice, Equal sweetener, and water in a large pitcher. Stir well until sweetener is dissolved.
2. Serve with ice.
3. Makes 6 servings.

Nutritional information (per glass):

Calories- 27, Fat- 0g, Carbohydrate- 6.8g, Protein- 0.1g, Sodium- 8g, and Total sugars- 4g.

Conclusion

Thank you again for purchasing the book Clean Eating Diet!

I am extremely excited to pass this information along to you, and I am so happy that you now have read and can hopefully implement these strategies going forward.

I hope this book was able to help you understand clean eating and other diet plans and how to use these diet plans to your advantage to lose weight and boost your metabolism.

The next step is to get started using this information and to hopefully live a healthier and happier life!

Please don't be someone who just reads this information and doesn't apply it, the strategies in this book will only benefit you if you use them!

If you know of anyone else that could benefit from the information presented here please inform them of this book.

Finally, if you enjoyed this book and feel it has added value to your life in any way, please take the time to share your thoughts and post a review on Amazon. It'd be greatly appreciated!

Thank you and good luck!

Preview Of:

Ultimate Coconut Oil Guide!

<u>Coconut Oil</u>

Coconut Oil Recipes For Organic Skin Care And Natural Beauty, Clean Eating For Weight Loss, Shinning Hair, Better Brain Function And Overall Health!

Introduction

I want to thank you and congratulate you for purchasing the book, *Coconut Oil: Ultimate Coconut Oil Guide! - Coconut Oil Recipes For Organic Skin Care And Natural Beauty, Clean Eating For Weight Loss, Shining Hair, Better Brain Function And Overall Health!*

This book contains proven steps and strategies on how you can take full advantage of the beauty, weight loss and health benefits that coconut oil has to offer. Through this book, you will learn more about:

- What makes coconut oil healthy?

- How it can help you get better, more glowing skin.

- Its effects on your hair and making healthier.

- Can coconut oil improve your brain function?

- Weight loss benefits and how it can boost your metabolism.

- Coconut oil and how it can help treat different illnesses.

- Recipes for both your diet as well as organic skin care.

- How to choose the right coconut oil for your needs.

We hope that through this book, you'll be able to recognize the amount of potential that a single bottle of coconut oil contains.

Thanks again for purchasing this book, I hope you enjoy it!

Chapter 1: Coconut Oil For Natural Beauty And Health

These days, more and more people are becoming aware of the effects that chemically manufactured products has on their bodies. As such, many of them have turned to a greener, more organic lifestyle that advocates going all natural when it comes to their food as well as the different products that they use on their bodies.

This isn't surprising, of course, considering the fact that there are a number of illnesses which are associated with constant use of synthetic and often chemical-laden skin and health products. There are certain risks that one must bear when using it; risks which can be avoided altogether if one were to switch over to something that's a bit closer to nature.

The coconut oil is a favorite among health buffs as it is one of those by-products that can be used in a multitude of ways. On one hand, it can be eaten and taken as a supplement which would boost your overall health. On the other, it can be applied topically and used as a beauty product as well as a means of treating certain skin issues.

You get all of these benefits but without worrying about its harmful effects to the body.

Why is it considered one of the best natural remedies out there?

It's all in the composition. About 99% of it is composed of saturated fats (which, in this case isn't as bad as it sounds) as well as traces of polyunsaturated fatty acids and monosaturated fatty acids. Virgin coconut oil retains a higher amount of the good stuff thus it is also valued higher.

It also contains lauric acid and quite a generous amount of it at that. When digested by the body, this would turn into monolaurin and is very beneficial when it comes to dealing with different bacteria and viruses. Diseases such as influenza and herpes are just two of the things that coconut oil can cure in a jiff. A tablespoon of it a day keeps the doctor away, so to speak.

Besides these, it is also one of the most powerful inhibitors of quite a number of different pathogenic organisms ranging from your usual viruses to even protozoa. All of this, of course, is attributed to its high lauric acid content.

For beauty and skincare

Coconut can also be used for cosmetic or skin care purposes. We'll get to the specifics of this in later chapters but to quickly summarize, it is often used for: Hair care, skin care, nails, lips as well as treating different skin issues such as psoriasis. It helps keep the skin youthful and glowing as well as protect it from harmful UV rays.

Thanks for Previewing My Exciting Book Entitled:

"Coconut Oil: Ultimate Coconut Oil Guide! Coconut Oil Recipes For Organic Skin Care And Natural Beauty, Clean Eating For Weight Loss, Shinning Hair, Better Brain Function And Overall Health!"

To purchase this book, simply go to the Amazon Kindle store and simply search:

"COCONUT OIL"

Then just scroll down until you see my book. You will know it is mine because you will see my name "Sarah Brooks" underneath the title.

Alternatively, you can visit my author page on Amazon to see this book and other work I have done. Thanks so much, and please don't forget your free bonuses

DON'T LEAVE YET! - CHECK OUT YOUR FREE BONUSES BELOW!

Free Bonus Offer: Get Free Access To The LiveFitVIP.com VIP Newsletter!

Once you enter your email address you will immediately get free access to this awesome newsletter!

But wait, right now if you join now for free you will also get free access to the "The 7 Keys To Body Transformation" free EBook!

To claim both your FREE VIP NEWSLETTER MEMBERSHIP and your FREE BONUS EBook on THE 7 KEYS TO BODY TRANSFORMATION!

Just Go To

www.liveFitVIP.com

www.ingramcontent.com/pod-product-compliance
Lightning Source LLC
Chambersburg PA
CBHW070937290526
45795CB00003B/1043